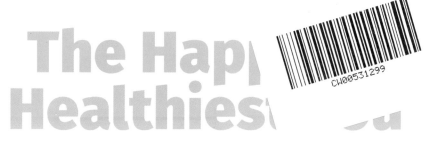

The Happier Healthiest You

The Missing Link To Feeling Great & Re-Discovering Your Mojo

10 Easy To Follow Steps To Get The Body & Mindset You Desire

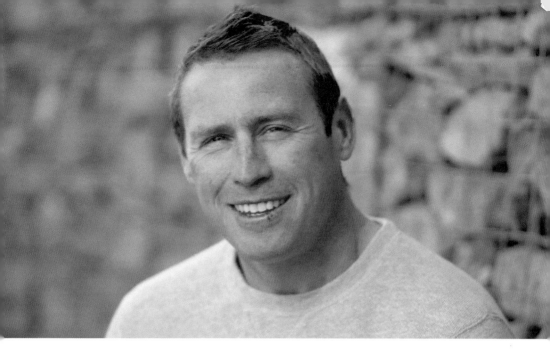

The Author

Damian is an expert in holistic health practices, focusing on nutrition, mindset, exercise and sleep to optimise overall health. He helps people become healthier and happier through human behaviour techniques and coaching to achieve their health and fitness goals.

He has been in the health and fitness industry for over 22 years, running Complete Personal Training in the heart of Dalkey for over 20 years.

With a background in coaching that spans back over 30 years, Damian is passionate about helping people "Put the pieces together" when it comes to health and wellness. With so much conflicting information out there, it's hard to know where to start.

He recognized the missing link between having an idea of what to do and what to eat, and then actually going and doing it consistently. This is where the 90 Day Body & Mindset Matrix™ was born.

"Master the mindset, and you'll never have to diet again." One of Damian's inspiration statements and the ethos that he lives by.

Having been a semi-professional rugby player for 15 years, and representing his country with the Irish Club and Irish Legends rugby team, he possesses a wealth of knowledge of what makes people tick, teamwork and what it takes to succeed on how to get to and through places that make you uncomfortable.

"There's no goal worth achieving that doesn't take some sort of sacrifice along the way"

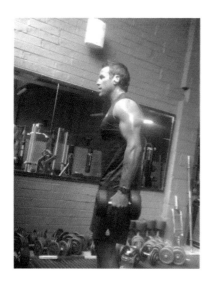
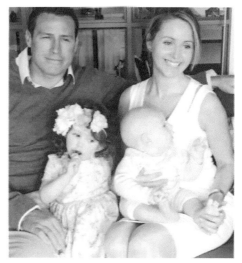
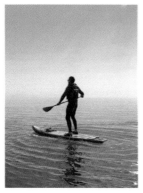
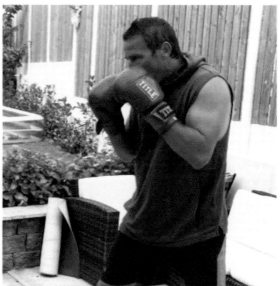
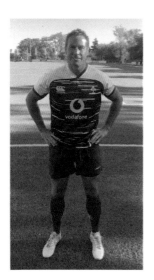
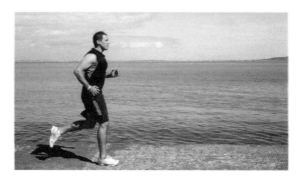

Introduction

Thanks for taking the time to read my first book. You have acquired it, that's great, but the biggest mistake people make is consume information and fail to act and implement it. But having bought it, it means you value your health and wellness and understand that you need to invest in it to get results. By invest, I mean time, effort, commitment and financially to have skin in the game, which is always a good motivator.

This book is designed to offer the reader a simple yet holistic approach to helping them reach optimal health and become the happiest healthiest version of themselves.

The book is not necessarily designed to read from front to back, you can pick out what interests you and put it all together as you see fit.

I like information explained to me in simple-terms, and I'd like to think I have done the same with this book. I have been thinking about writing this book for over 10 years, and have finally gotten around to writing it. I hope you enjoy it.

Our Why

My team and I just love helping people just like you, to get your mojo back and get back to the happiest healthiest version of you. It lights me up seeing the happiness and confidence find its way back as seen by the glint in your eyes as you find something that actually works and is sustainable. You see, we work with you on your mindset, the one thing that has been holding you back for so long. Learning about diet and exercise is one thing, consistently doing it is another thing altogether, and that's what you've been struggling with right?

Let's dive in.

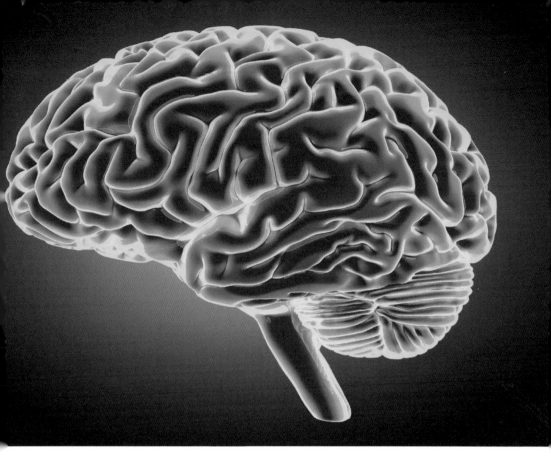

The Brain

When it comes to changing from current to desired behaviours, understanding how your brain works is a great place to start.

What is the role of the brain?

The role of the brain is to keep you alive, that's it. Nothing more, nothing less.

It understands the difference between danger and safety but not reality and make believe. It issues a fight or flight response when in danger and takes you away from danger or will help you fight the danger. It will always try and help you get to safety to keep you alive.

How the brain is a series of Loops

The brain works in a series of loops. It receives information, it filters the information and puts meaning or interpretation to it. Then there's an output i.e. a behaviour. This process is the one that is often overlooked when trying to change. Most people look to just change the output without addressing the previous loops, which means you are fighting a losing battle, sound familiar?

How we filter information

The reticular activating system filters the incoming information which quite often can become overly negative, where we filter out a lot of positives and focus on the negatives. If you are feeling negative, and air on the side of pessimism, you have literally trained it to take out the positives and focus on the negatives. When we are tending to filter in the negatives, this affects every other loop i.e. the interpretation and output. This means that the meaning or perception we attach to the information we've just processed through our filter is more negative and then the output or behaviour becomes more negative as a result.

The key to change is to altering the filtering process of the reticular activating system. By doing this, we change the rest of the series of loops of the brain. We can do this by firstly setting out what you want to achieve, and where you would like to be in 365 days, in terms of how you would like to look, behave and think. Then we need to work out how we are going to get there.

To help with the filtering process, we need to start sharing our wins each and every day. By doing this, we train our brain to look for and seek out more wins which changes the filtering process over to positives rather than negatives. This is turn, as I mentioned, changes the rest of the loop process (remember the filter -> interpretation -> output?) which organically changes your behaviours to more positive ones.

What are our subconscious and conscious roles?

Think of our Conscious mind being the captain steering the ship in the right direction, and the subconscious being the crew putting the work in moving and getting places in the direction it's been told (for the most part).

The problem is, some of the crew members are pulling in the direction that they were told, when they were younger, was in the best interest of the ship (i.e. you), but now that we are older and wiser, these behaviours or that direction the crew member is pulling us in, no longer serves us in the best way.

Think about it, treating yourself with food and mindless eating at the weekend are just two examples.

You were given a treat when you were good when you were a child. Now as an adult, when you do something well, you immediately turn to food to celebrate as a "treat", a learned behaviour. Similarly, at the weekends your parents may have got a takeaway or given you a nicer cereal, or pocket money to buy sweets, we are now doing the adult version of that learned behaviour, with adult foods and drinks.

But they aren't serving you particularly well right?

You think you can't change, but you can, it's just that you are committed to this behaviour as it's been engrained from an early age.

The critical faculty, (say what?)

In the early years all the way up to the age of 9, you are learning your map of reality, uploading your brain's software, personalities and your view of how the world works. At this age, you don't have a subconscious, you just do and say what you like, with no filter or consequence for your actions.

It's only when you reach the age of 9, the subconscious develops, and what you have learned and the way you see the world to date is what your brain deems to be what it's happy to move forward with, as the best strategy to keep you alive (it's main job right?).

Your subconscious develops and with this, the critical faculty develops, which serves as a security guard for all the information including your view of how the world works, map of reality and your learned behaviours and map of reality.

And it's locked in...

The critical faculty takes its job extremely seriously, and won't let these learned behaviours change easily, unless either one of these two things happen.

You imagine, or you emote. So in simple terms, you imagine something or a scenario or you strongly feel an emotion. By doing this, you lower the critical faculties guard, making you more suggestible to change and the re-programming of your initial map of realities etc.

Pretty cool right?

This is where hypnotherapy can really help. It sounds very out there because we've all seen the shows on TV, but that's not what real hypnotherapy represents. It can be a non-trance variation where you use your imagination to tap into the subconscious to make permanent changes towards desired behaviours, like making better decisions that will serve you better.

Synopsis

The brain works in a series of loops

It's main job is to keep you safe and alive

Your reticular activating system filters information as you consume it

You then put meaning to the information and interpret it

The critical faculty protects your map of reality once your subconscious has formed at the age of 8-9

Non trance hypnosis (that I am trained in) is a great way to change behaviours

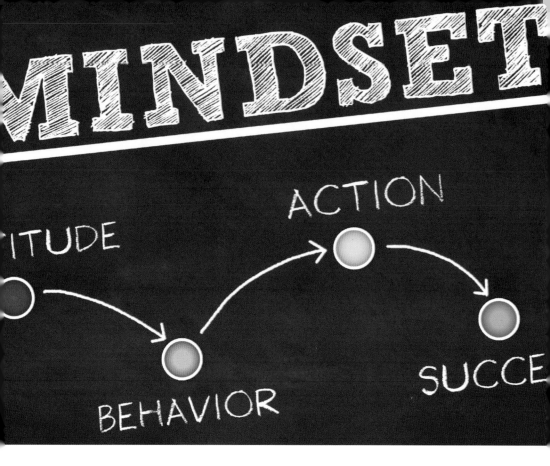

MINDSET

ITUDE → BEHAVIOR → ACTION → SUCCE

Your Mindset

Being able to understand how your mindset works and, more importantly, having control over your feelings is pretty important when making long term changes. Remember eating that tub of ice cream when you were upset?

So when you have a thought, it can soon become a feeling and manifest into a longer term mood that may last until you do something about it, unless you understand the process of how to change the initial thought and stop it at source so to speak.

There are several ways to do this.

Change your physiology - Exercise in any form or meditation/ breath work

Change your state - Journal for gratitude (write down 3-5 things you are grateful for)

A pattern interrupt - Interrupt the thought pattern (listen to your favourite song or watch something that makes you laugh)

The above are very simple exercises you can do that cost nothing, but are you prepared to do them if you have a negative thought?

[Maybe, but] That is one of the keys to avoid falling into the negative feeling or negative mood that can start with just one negative thought and spiral.

The other way we can do this is to change the reticular activating system or the filtering process that decides how information goes into our brain a mentioned in the previous chapter.

Why do we self-sabotage?

This is a largely common behaviour in the health and wellness space. When we talked about the brain's job to keep us safe and alive in previous chapters, we have to understand that the brain doesn't know the difference of you being fit or unfit, skinny, overweight, happy or unhappy.

As we mentioned before, its perogative is to keep you alive, nothing else.

We also know it is predictive; it predicts the future from what has happened before and current inputs to predict the future and your future behaviours, so as far as it knows, it's doing a great job keeping you alive (it's one and only job, it doesn't care if you are fit/unfit/happy/sad etc.).

This is why the Monday morning diet doesn't work, nor does the one you've tried before and failed over and over again.

So the brain does not really like change very much especially when you try and do things differently or make a BIG deal of the changes, as it's uncharted waters it doesn't recognise.

It says NO to change and sends in the negative ego to talk you out of the different behaviour you are showing i.e. in diet changes, starting to exercise. The negative ego will tell you to "eat the cake", "stay on the couch", justifying it for you in the mean-time.

What's the negative ego or the saboteur?

So the negative ego is there to keep you alive. It's doing the job of the critical faculty (remember the security guard?) and the brain. It's sitting on your shoulder telling you what you should or shouldn't do, according to the story you've been telling yourself for so many years, that has now become your reality, and is the main reason you find yourself in your current place in your life.

Wherever you are and whatever you are doing in your life, is largely down to the story you have been telling yourself for your whole life that is:-

A) Limiting your beliefs

B) Putting YOU in the way of your own progress

C) In control of your decision making

How can I control my inner monologue?

Controlling this voice can be challenging but is doable. We talked about this in earlier chapters in terms of filtering information and interpreting information. We also mentioned being able to change your state and your physiology through breath work, asking yourself certain questions, journaling, gratitude and pattern interrupts.

Catching your negative thoughts that come from your negative ego, before they turn into feelings, is important to prevent the negative thought from turning into a negative day, week or month

When you are looking to change your behaviours, you've got to try and fly under the radar so to speak. Try not to make it a big deal in your head. So what I mean by that is, try and be blasé about the changes you are about to make, do it quietly without fuss.

Your brain doesn't like change, so it will be very reluctant unless you sneak it past your negative ego and minimise the disruption in your life and in your head. When making the changes to the filtering process, such as sharing your wins, expect there to be times when your negative ego has something negative to say and tells you it's not worth it, it's not working, go drink the wine, stay on the couch, to try and keep you in the same place.

Why, because what it's done in the past has been spot on as far as it's concerned. It's kept you alive right? Job done. But that's not enough or you wouldn't be reading this book.

And it shouldn't be enough, you deserve the best version of you, and so do the people around you.

What's your old story?

Understand that your thoughts are perceptive based. They are not reality. In fact, pretty much everything you think about could be questioned in terms of it being true. Your thoughts are simply the interpretation you have put to something you have seen, heard, or thought about.

So in simple terms, the thoughts you have been telling yourself for five, ten even fifty years, are now your reality. The story you have been telling yourself for however long is now something you are committed to, because that's how you believe the world works and your perception of it.

What comes with this is your commitment to the behaviour that has become your reality. You truly believe that this is the best way forward for you, but in fact the current story you tell yourself is most likely the thing that is limiting your beliefs and keeping you stuck in the same pattern of behaviours.

How can I build the new story I want?

Identifying your old story and understanding how you speak to yourself on a daily basis can be a fascinating insight to what generally turns out to be a pretty consistent road map of the direction your life takes in terms of consistent daily actions. Cumulatively, these actions take you in a direction at a pretty fast speed, but is it the direction you desire?

Building the story that you want to become your reality is where you need to start when it comes to changing behaviours. It takes time and it takes daily consistency. When building out the new story, it's crucial to have a direction that you want your life to take. What do you want the new story to be and what do you want the desired outcome to be.

How do you imagine your way to the desired results?

Your brain and mindset is the most powerful tool you possess. Master these, and it will bring you a more fulfilling, less stressful, happier and healthier life.

Being able to imagine or emote to reduce the critical faculty we mentioned in the previous chapters is the first port of call. Let's use imagination as it's a little easier to control.

So, close your eyes and imagine yourself in 365 day's time.

> What do you look like?
> How do you feel?
> Where are you?
> How do the clothes you want to wear feel?
> What's the weather like?

Can you see that picture clearly in your head? You now have to imagine that outcome as many times a day as you can. The importance of this can't be underestimated, you see your brain doesn't know the difference between real and make believe. So the more you can imagine 'YOU' down the line, the more your brain will magnetically pull you towards the desired behaviours that will get you to your desired outcome.

Part of your daily mindset exercises should be to set your intentions each and every day consistently for at least 1000 repetitions so you go from what's called a cognitive behaviour (have to think about doing it) to an autonomous (automatic) one. Yes it takes this long, so strap yourself in, get comfortable and be prepared to be consistent to create an autonomous behaviour.

What are affirmations and how can they help?

When you are building out your new story, using affirmations as an extra form of self-communication is a massively powerful tool in helping you reach your desired outcome. Affirmations are simply telling yourself in your head, saying them out loud, reading them or listening to whatever it is you want to achieve. This is similar and in complete alignment with imagining the outcomes and visualization.

You are most suggestible to new ideas first thing in the morning and last thing at night before you go to sleep. These are the ideal times to listen to and say your affirmations which are in alignment with the desired outcome i.e. I want to be more confident, I want to fit into a size x dress, I want to feel more relaxed etc. Visualising, listening to, or thinking about the desired outcome more often or as many times a day as you can, will help trick your brain into thinking that this is a reality. This will help pull your behaviour towards the desired outcome.

Don't underestimate the power of visualisation, affirmations, and imagining that outcome.

Synopsis

Negative thoughts are normal, try not to let them linger

Change your state, physiology through journaling, breath work and pattern interrupt

The negative ego is sent in to sabotage you when trying new behaviours

Use visualisation to imagine the outcome you want

Affirmations are when you tell yourself who you want to be, what you want & when you want it to make it happen

Your old story is what you've been telling yourself for so long that it has become your reality

You can build out your new story to be whatever you want it to be. You just need to consistently tell yourself the new story

You are most suggestible to new ideas and behaviours first thing in the morning or last thing at night

1,000 reps of your mindset exercises will change your behaviour to go from cognitive to autonomous

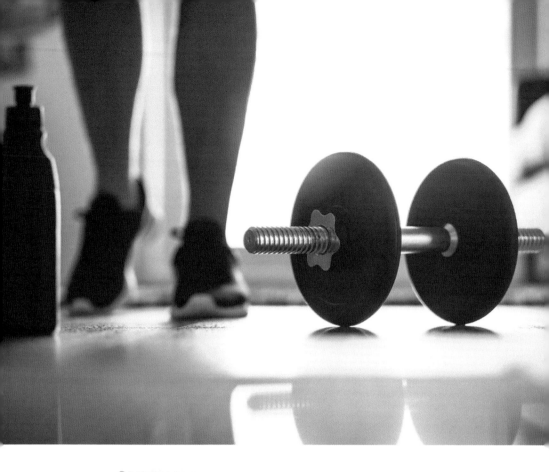

Exercise

Exercise is the first port of call when it comes to living a balanced, happy and healthy lifestyle, physically and mentally. You hear people talking about releasing those amazing Endorphins, but this is a real thing. Have you ever finished a workout and thought "Why did I do that?" "I regret that bit of exercise". The short answer is no.

Exercise is the first port of call when it comes to living a balanced, happy and healthy lifestyle, physically and mentally. You hear people talking about releasing those amazing Endorphins, but this a real thing. Have you ever finished a workout and thought "Why did I do that?" "I regret that bit of exercise". The short answer is no.

It's one of the best mood lifters, state changers and gifts we were given. It should be something you appreciate rather than dread. The key to that is finding something you enjoy doing.

Whilst the feeling before you exercise is quite often not in alignment with the feeling you know you will get after it, it's something to keep in the back of your mind when procrastinating before-hand.

That's where several factors come in

Accountability

Community

Enjoyment

Progress

Results

Without the above, it can be a tough battle against your negative ego to get out and just do it. You know the voice that justifies not going to exercise and tries to give you a perfectly good excuse to stay put on the couch or at your desk i.e. "I'll do it tomorrow" or "It's starting to rain". Sound familiar?

Understanding the vast array of benefits that exercise will give you is not to be under estimated. Below is just a few of them.

- Helps improve mood

- Helps mental health disorders and our ability to help deal with all the stressors that today's world throws at us

- Reduces anxiety

- Reduces body fat levels

- Helps you move better

- Gets you stronger

- Helps you carry out daily movements/activities far more efficiently

- Helps increase muscle mass to boost metabolism

- Improves cardio vascular health

- Increases blood flow and arterial health

- Lowers bad cholesterol

- Lowers blood pressure

- Improves bone strength and density

- Increases energy levels

- Improves sleep

- Improves the absorption of amino acids (protein)

Pretty cool list of amazing things right? Now let's get you moving. Find something you enjoy. This could be something you used to do and stopped or something you haven't tried and have been meaning to. Or, it could be something as simple as meeting a friend for a walk and a chat.

What's the best time/type?

There's no best time to exercise, it's a completely personal preference that is up to the individual and the logistics involved. I personally like to exercise in the morning as I feel amazing for the day and have a lovely sense of achievement for the day, not to mention, allowing you to eat a few extra calories is always nice.

How mobility and flexibility will enhance my life?

Daily stretching will help release muscle tension and reduce the pull on your joints, which in turn will help reduce tension, helping joints move more freely. By doing this, you will reduce the risk of osteoarthritis and other muscular and joint injuries.

Taking joints through their full range of motion on a daily basis will help with muscle memory and improving synovial fluid production, helping reduce friction and increasing lubrication of the joint.

Why you must use resistance?

When you hear of resistance training or weight training, you might think of Arnold Schwarzenegger's rippling muscles and be a little put off by the concept. Firstly, this is not a likely outcome, because you are not pumping yourself full of growth hormone and anabolic steroids. If you are a female reading this, you don't produce enough testosterone to grow muscles like Arnie.

The fact is, aesthetics are only a small part of lifting weights or resistance bands or even just using your body weight. To prevent osteoporosis, increase your calorie burn and help you live a long healthy pain free life I would recommend the Complete Nutrition System and Complete Afterburn workouts.

Why do cardio?

Increasing your heart rate in any form can be considered cardio. I'm not a big fan of monotonous steady state cardio as I find it a little boring. I like to put some resistance exercises together to help make your heart rate go up, or play a sport that takes your mind off the fitness aspect i.e. chasing a ball or concentrating on winning a game.

Jogging, rowing, cycling or swimming in a straight line for a long period doesn't appeal to me, but that doesn't in any way mean it is any less beneficial for you. It's just personal preference.

As I mentioned before, anything that gets your heart rate up is beneficial for you, and the more you enjoy it, the more you are likely to do it. So in my opinion, that's your perfect cardio choice, the one you are going to partake in.

Depending on your body type, you will be more suited to a certain energy system (uses different sources of fuel for energy) or specific type of training. For example, you see a specific sprinter shape versus a marathon runner shape. A marathon runner would not make a great sprinter and a great sprinter will not make a good marathon runner. You are either one or the other or somewhere inbetween.

The likelihood is, you are somewhere in between.

You might have a slightly better 'engine' to perform longer distance cardio or marathon running with slow twitch muscle fibres (usually an Ectomorph), or better at the explosive, higher impact, high intensity interval training or heavy weighted exercises where you would be considered more suited to sprinting (usually a Mesomorph).

If you are good at something or enjoy one type of exercise more i.e. better at longer steady state cardio or you like pushing yourself and prefer high intensity training then do what you enjoy. The likelihood is you will do it more and progress further in a shorter amount of time.

Synopsis

Exercise helps you live longer in the majority of cases

Cardio can be in any form that gets your heart rate up

Do the cardio version you enjoy

Use resistance to enhance your life, burn more calories, prevent osteoporosis, carry out day to day activities more efficiently

Exercise will always leave you with a sense of achievement, feel good factor, a clear head, and some "you" time and can break a cycle of negative thoughts and emotions

Incorporate mobility and flexibility to relieve joint pain, reduce joint friction improve overall body movement

Join a community, team, training gym that gives you accountability, support, affirmation, access and attention like our members get at Complete Personal Training

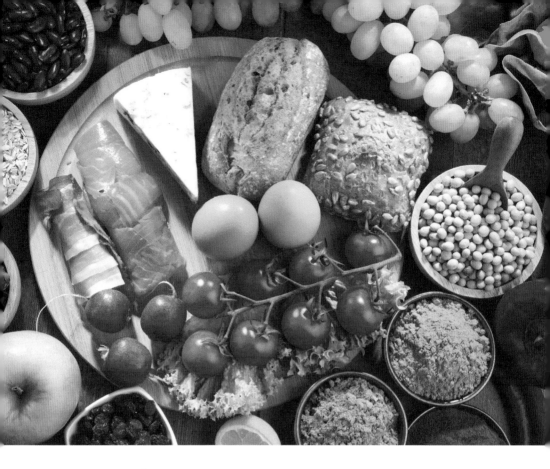

Nutrition

One of the most under-estimated forms of health. What you put into your body will either nourish or poison it. A quote I really like is:-

"Food can be the most effective form of medicine or the slowest form of poison".

This is so true, as it may not cause you to get sick in 1 year or 30 years, but at some point, the food you have chosen to consume over the period of your life will have a massive bearing on your health and wellness.

How does food affect me?

Food will energise you or drain you. Most people just accept where they are on the energy scale and that's the hand they are dealt.

NO.

The food you eat and the way you choose to live your life, will determine your energy levels, your mood, how your body functions and even your mental health, which I will explain in our gut health chapter.

Are all calories equal?

In my opinion and backed up by research the effect of food on hormones, on your cell make up and the make-up of how well your body functions will be determined equally by quality and quantity of the calories you consume. It is true that you are what you eat. Your body regenerates every 6 months or so.

So if you've been eating processed, synthetic foods...your body performance will reflect that.

However, if you are eating clean, one ingredient foods as close to their natural state as possible, your energy, mental clarity and overall quality of life will reflect that. Eating fresh fruit and veg, good quality meat and fish, with the right anti-inflammatory grains and dairy added, will have you firing on all cylinders, keeping toxicity low and nourishing your body with all the nutrients, fibre and quality calories it needs to thrive.

When coaching my clients, I always start with working on the quality of the calories eaten. I start with this, as it matters just as much as the quantity.

The fundamentals of getting and staying healthy in terms of nutrition is a combination of:-

A) Energy balance i.e. calories in versus calories out. Are you eating less than you are burning if you are looking at losing weight?

B) The quality of calories you are consuming

If you can get the balance right, then you can do nothing but lose weight. Now there are plenty of moving parts to this, because hormones, medication, metabolic damage and gut health all have an effect on the speed and consistency of weight loss.

Macro nutrients in simple terms

Protein

- It helps us build muscle

- It helps us feel fuller for longer

- It takes the most calories to burn when digesting (burning calories when eating is pretty cool right?)

- Most of your meals should be based around this macro nutrient

- Good sources are whole eggs, fresh fish, good quality chicken, red meat and edamame beans

Fat

- Your body needs fats to survive and function properly

- Your body needs most types of fat to function optimally

- The only fat we shouldn't be consuming is Trans fats (the nasty ones that are chemically altered through processing at high heat)

- Man makes bad fats, nature does not

- When I say eat fat, embrace them, and yes I mean all natural fats - Saturated (animal fats and coconut oil from unprocessed sources), Polyunsaturated (Eggs, Seeds, Fish, Omega 3's), Monounsaturated Fats (Olive oil, Nuts, Avocados)

- A combination of these Fats should be consumed in a ratio of 33% for optimal health

- Fats don't make you fat, over eating and making poor calorie choices does

- They contribute to a vast amount of bodily functions such as Heart and Brain function, Hair, Skin and Nails, balancing hormones, boosting metabolism and improving satiety levels

Fibres

- They perform massively important roles within the body

- It helps us regulate our gut and keep it functioning properly

- The vitamins and antioxidants present in these foods are awesome too

- These come in the form of nuts, seeds, green veg and certain grains

- You can get all the fibre you need without having to consume grains

- Get the majority of fibre from whole fruits, vegetables and nuts/seed
- Better choice for all round quality and bang for your buck than grains

Carbohydrates
- This is the one macronutrient that your body doesn't actually need (sorry)
- Carbohydrates, consumed in any form, will be broken down to sugar eventually, depending on the type
- If you eat a high sugar food = a fast releasing carbohydrate which increases your blood sugars immediately
- Eating sugary foods or indeed foods high in carbohydrate with every meal can be detrimental to reaching optimal health
- For the most part, we are consuming too many carbohydrates making us addicted to the initial dopamine hit we get after consuming them
- The source you should choose is both anti-inflammatory and high in fibre (things like sweet potato, Basmati rice, Buckwheat).
- Your body tolerates the higher sugar foods/carbohydrate straight after intense exercise

Let's address Carbohydrates first. They're not evil and have a place in your diet. We just have an issue in over consumption of them. The problem is, we eat Carbs, then we can't stop eating them and end up over eating on calories.

Just like Carbohydrates, fats have been vilified in the past. Make no mistake, fats are crucial for the body to function properly. Heart, brain, skin, nails, cells and the rest. So going low fat is going to take you further away from optimal health and wellness, rather than what you may have been told in the past.

There is no such thing as a bad natural fat, man-made fats are the ones you want to avoid. Fats that have had their molecular structure changed through high heat and chemical additions. Fats such as trans fats can have massive inflammatory effect on your body. These types of fats are used to keep foods for longer and make them seem tasty and more palatable, not to mention being cheap fillers for food companies.

When trying to lose weight, a really good place to start is working out how many calories you should be consuming, then aiming to be under that by about 200-300 calories. You can work out how many calories you require to lose, maintain or gain weight on my website www.completepersonaltraining.ie. My fitness pal is a good place to input your calories, once you have figured out how many you need to reach your desired outcome.

What's the best eating plan for me?

The best eating plan for you, is the one that you can manage long term. Initially if there are gut issues, an exclusion diet (taking certain foods out) is required to give your gut a chance to recover and heal.

Other than that, the quality and quantity of calories is the best place to start. I wouldn't be worrying too much about how much fat, protein or carbs you are consuming, at least until you have the fundamentals in place.

However, once you have zoomed in on these, depending on your body type (remember Ectomorph, Endomorph and Mesomorph?), I would recommend slight differences in your macro nutrient consumption

Ectomorph - Thin, wiry, fast metabolism, can generally eat what they want. Finds it hard to put on weight.
Recommended Macro Break down - Carbs 60% Protein 20% Fats 20%

Endomorph - Thicker set, puts on muscle easily. Puts on weight easily, finds it hard to lose it..
Recommended Macro Break down - Carbs 10% Protein 30% Fats 60%

Mesomorph - Athletic build. Puts on muscle easily. Naturally low body fat
Recommended Macro Break down - Carbs 40% Protein 30% Fats 30%

Find what works for you. I for one, am the latter i.e. fat works for me as I'm an endomorph. Fat sky rockets my energy and concentration and keeps me lean, carbs send me to sleep.

The Complete Nutrition System™

Please Note: This is a system for lifestyle change not a diet. Think about the way you want to live as opposed to the diet plan you are on. I have spent 20 years tweaking and developing this system to help get you to your optimal health. If you put the Complete Nutrition System™ contents into practice, this information will change your life in terms of increasing mental clarity, energy levels, mood and general wellbeing.

Before you can achieve maximum fat loss, optimum health should be your main goal. Getting your gut health/immune system and hormones functioning optimally are all massively important before optimum body composition can be achieved.

The main point is to KISS (Keep It Simple Stupid). The closest 'Diet' term I can give to my Complete Nutrition System™ is 'Paleo with a twist'. The Complete Nutrition System™ is based on eating one ingredient foods as close to their natural states as possible! This is an anti-inflammatory eating plan. When we eat foods we can't tolerate, they cause an immune response, by your body promoting inflammation (joint pain/brain fog/anxiety/illness).

Anti-inflammatory grains such as Quinoa, Basmati Rice, Sweet potato, Potato, Gluten Free Oats and Buckwheat are recommended **POST TRAINING ONLY**, meaning we are not craving them or as restricted like the Paleo diet. We recommend goats and sheep dairy but not cows dairy, because of the loss of digestive enzymes needed to digest by humans through the chemicals used during processing cow's dairy.

What do I eat and when?

When it comes to nutrient timing, I'm a firm believer in refuelling after your workout with Carbohydrates. This is the time when your energy (glycogen) stores are most open and (tolerant of) carbohydrates and refuelling for your next workout. This works really well and will have you fired up and ready for your next workout even if you don't have much food before it.

Post workout

So your post workout meal should consist of carbs to refuel and protein to build muscle and recover for the most part.

Any time meal

Your any time meals should be lower in carbohydrate as you don't need to be refuelled and you don't want to spike your blood sugar levels as this will promote fat storage and make fat loss a slower process. Your blood sugars are spiked by taking in a carbohydrate. All carbohydrates will turn to sugar at some stage but the slower releasing ones (such as oats, sweet potato etc) will have less effect on your blood sugar levels. Fibre is generally the reason foods have higher or lower effects on your blood sugar levels.

This meal should consist more of fibrous vegetables, proteins and fats. Fats and proteins will have far less effect on your blood sugar levels.

Pre workout

Eating a low Carbohydrate snack pre training with more fat and some protein will give you more of a balanced energy level especially when it comes to fat loss. You see, if you give your body sugar for fuel pre workout, what do you think it's preferred source of fuel will be? Yes, sugar, so the thought process behind this is, reduce carbs before your workout and refuel with them after the workout for your next workout where you will have full glycogen stores.

This meal should consist more of fibrous vegetables, proteins and fats. Fats and proteins will have far less effect on your blood sugar levels, similar to your anytime meal.

Cows Dairy

- It's highly processed and the digestive enzyme needed to digest it is absent in humans

Wheat and Gluten

- The majority of humans have intolerances to wheat and gluten which, as a result, causes inflammation, water retention, brain fuzz and lethargy

Sugar

- Fructose (fruit sugar is ok in its whole fruit form, reduce juices) Lactose (dairy sugar, ok in small amounts in goats and sheep form) Sucrose (table sugar - reduce refined sugar). Additives, preservative, flavourings, colourings,

Meal prep

Meal prep is the difference between you sticking to a plan and not. While you are working on making your new habits permanent i.e. making your cognitive behaviours autonomous, it is crucial to be prepared for at least the next 3 meals ahead i.e. know what you are going to eat 3 meals ahead.

Here are some top tips to helping you get there:-

- Planning and preparation is the key and the difference to your dietary success or failure

- Use Sunday and Wednesday as your preparation days to bulk cook and prepare meals. Prepare from Monday to Wednesday and Wednesday to Sunday

- Don't go shopping when you are hungry

- Don't let yourself get hungry

- Sometimes we have to grab a quick bite so below are some good snack ideas

Snacks

1. Celery sticks with a nut butter to fill to the hollow portion. My favorites being cashew

2. Dried meats. I really like biltong

3. Celery with goats cheese

4. Canned Tuna

5. Chocolate/Strawberry protein smoothie with frozen berries/green veg

6. Branched chain amino acid powder and essential amino acid powder. I really like to drink this when I go to the gym

7. Turkey or roast beef slices rolled into dark greens, a.k.a. high protein roll-ups. The green used, like kale or spinach, provides a more pleasant taste to the palate and of course fiber

8. Haloumi cheese and olives

9. Hard boiled eggs and cashews

10. Berries and Almonds (Almonds fried in coconut oil sprinkled with smoked paprika)

Hydration

Imagine you are a camel and heading out to the desert for a couple of days. Your body will fill up with water and save it in its humps as a reservoir for the drought ahead.

You as a human, are the same (you are a camel). You literally are in an emergency storage mode as your body is terrified it's going to run out, so stores it.

Drink more water (2-3 Litres per day) combined with taking out inflammatory foods.

Watch your body rid itself of excess water

WHY?

- Because your body needs it for optimal health
- If your body is starved of water it retains it
- It detoxes and flushes toxins out of your body
- A dehydrated body won't perform, even 1% dehydrated will affect performance
- If you can't work out properly, you won't get the best possible results
- Every bodily function is reliant on water to function optimally

Synopsis

Eat natural one ingredient nutrient dense foods as close to their natural state as possible

Make protein and vegetables the base of most of your meals

Embrace fat, your body needs it

Consume less sugary foods and replace with better quality carbohydrates

Drink more quality water (2 litres)

Eat your main carb feed after intense exercise

Take fish Oils, probiotics and Vitamin D3 and Apple Cider Vinegar

Be patient, bodies take time to change.

Don't obsess with the scales, some weeks you WILL NOT LOSE WEIGHT

This is a Marathon/Lifestyle not a sprint/diet

Supplement your diet with green powder and fish oil (2-3 grams per day)

There is no end to being healthy. Treat your eating plan as something you will be doing from now on. Find foods you love and start from there. Build out your recipe from there.

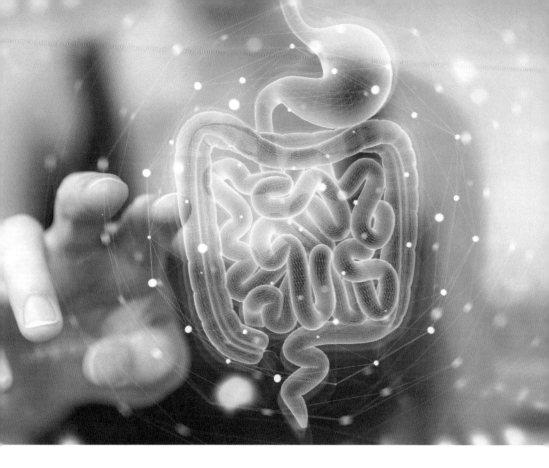

Gut Health

The gut is not something you would ever think of having such an important role within the body's phenomenal interior. It not only helps you absorb the nutrients you've consumed, but it also plays a massive factor in your mental health.

Yup, sounds odd, but hear me out.

It plays such an important role within the body that it is often referred to as the second brain. To take it one step further, I'm a firm believer that if your gut is not functioning properly, it is likely your brain isn't either.

The gut has been researched more and more over the last decade. The reality has become clear that it has more roles within overall health than we ever imagined. Up until a few years ago, the gut was considered a simple long tube for our food to pass through and be excreted.

What is the gut microbiome?

The term Gut Microbiome refers to the 300 to 500 types of bacteria and microorganisms living in our digestive tract. Although some can be harmful, for the most part, they have massively important roles to play in creating optimal health.

Who could have imagined the gut was largely responsible for immune system, mood, mental health, auto-immune disease, endocrine disorders, skin conditions, and even cancer. Bacteria line your intestine and help you digest food. They also send signals to the immune system and make small molecules that can help your brain function. You get gut flora at birth from your mother, but after that it's heavily influenced by lifestyle and eating habits.

What is inflammation and how does it affect me?

This eating plan is all about reducing foods that causes inflammation. Inflammation occurs in the gut. If you have chronic inflammation it has been linked to an increase in the chance of illness and disease. Reducing foods that cause inflammation is crucial on your journey to reach optimal health and fat loss.

5 Signs of an unhealthy gut

Skin Disorders - rashes, acne and dry skin, for the most part, can be traced back to an inability of the gut to tolerate a certain food or, where your endocrine system (in charge of hormones) is regulated.

Upset Stomach - when you eat certain foods and you have loose bowels or constant flatulence, look at what the constant is in your diet or take a note of what you eat and how you feel after each meal. Reactions to eating certain foods will generally be obvious, so the exclusion method is a great way to figure this out. We will cover this later in the chapter.

A high sugar diet - eating a lot of sugar in your diet will have adverse effects on your gut, especially the processed refined sugar that we just don't tolerate very well. It can cause inflammation which will damage your gut bacteria, also the negative spiral of sugar cravings and more likely more sugar and more gut damage.

Disturbed Sleep - Who would have thought sleep can have an effect on your gut. Lethargy. Serotonin the hormone that affects sleep and mood is produced in the gut. If the production is affected, this can affect your sleep especially sleep depth, causing chronic fatigue.

Autoimmune conditions - Did you know that the majority of your immune system resides in your gut? Inflammation is an immune response that causes your body to attack itself rather than attack external invaders. Reducing inflammatory factors through your lifestyle is a massive step forward in reaching optimal health. This can be where you live, what you eat, drink, inhale, absorb in your skin, wash your clothes with, wash yourself with.

The gut has a direct link to your brain via the vagus nerve, so when your gut is below par, it has direct communication to your brain, potentially causing anxiety, mood swings, brain fog (ever felt tired after a bowl of pasta or pizza) and, in extreme cases, depression. We have taken out the main culprits (wheat, gluten, cow's dairy) that affect the majority, as part of the Complete Nutrition System. I encourage you to remove wheat and gluten for an extended period, no less than 90 days, so you can allow the gut to heal and you will have more of a chance to be able to re-introduce them in the future.

7 things you can do for your gut health

1. **Lower your stress levels**

   Chronic high levels of stress are hard on your whole body, including your gut. Some ways to lower stress may include meditation, walking, getting a massage, spending time with friends or family, diffusing essential oils, decreasing caffeine intake, laughing, yoga, or having a pet.

2. **Get enough sleep**

   Not getting enough, or a sufficient quality of sleep, can have a serious impact on your gut health, which can in turn contribute to more sleep issues. Try to prioritize getting at least 7-8 hours of uninterrupted sleep per night. Your doctor may be able to help if you have trouble sleeping.

3. **Eat slowly**

   Chewing your food thoroughly and eating your meals more slowly can help promote full digestion and absorption of nutrients. This may help you reduce digestive discomfort and maintain a healthy gut.

4. Stay hydrated

Drinking plenty of water has been shown to have a beneficial effect on the mucosal lining of the intestines, as well as on the balance of good bacteria in the gut. Staying hydrated is a simple way to promote a healthy gut.

5. Take a prebiotic or probiotic

Adding a prebiotic and Probiotic supplement to your diet may be a great way to improve your gut health. Prebiotics provide "food" meant to promote the growth of beneficial bacteria in the gut, while probiotics are live good bacteria. People with bacterial overgrowth, such as SIBO, should not take probiotics. Not all probiotic supplements are high quality or will actually provide benefit. It's best to consult your healthcare provider when choosing a probiotic or prebiotic supplement to ensure the best health benefit.

6. Check for food intolerances

If you have symptoms such as cramping, bloating, abdominal pain, diarrhoea, rashes, nausea, fatigue, and acid reflux, you may be suffering from a food intolerance. You can try eliminating common trigger foods to see if your symptoms improve. If you are able to identify a food or foods that are contributing to your symptoms, you may see a positive change in your digestive health by changing your eating habits.

7. Change your diet

Reducing the amount of processed, high-sugar, and high-fat foods that you eat can contribute to better gut health. Additionally, eating plenty of plant-based foods and lean protein can positively impact your gut. A diet high in fibre has been shown to contribute tremendously to a healthy gut microbiome.

Four types of food to enhance your gut health

Diet and gut health are very closely linked. Avoiding processed foods, highly processed fat, and foods high in refined sugars is extremely important to maintaining a healthy microbiome, as these foods destroy good bacteria and promote growth of damaging bacteria. There are also a number of foods you can eat that actively promote the growth of beneficial bacteria, contributing to your overall health. These foods include:

1. **High-fibre foods**

   High fibre foods such as beans, peas, oats, bananas, berries, asparagus, avocados, chia seeds, broccoli and leeks have shown a positive impact on gut health in numerous studies.

2. **Prebiotics**

   Prebiotics are a source of food for your gut's healthy bacteria. They are carbohydrates your body can't digest. So they go to your lower digestive tract, where they act like food to help the healthy bacteria grow. Good examples of these would be cacao, garlic and onion which have great prebiotic cultures that are great for your digestion and serve to enhance your digestive process.

3. **Fermented foods (probiotics)**

   Fermented foods such as kimchi, sauerkraut, yogurt, tempeh, miso, and kefir are great dietary sources of probiotics. While the quality of these foods may vary, their benefits on the gut microbiome are well trusted resources. I would always recommend taking a high quality probiotic especially when you are embarking on your health and fitness journey.

4. **Collagen-boosting foods**

   Collagen-rich foods such as bone broth and salmon may be

beneficial to overall health and gut health specifically. Many of these benefits are anecdotal conclusions and further research will be done. You could also try to boost your body's own collagen production through foods. Try adding a variety of foods, like mushrooms, good sheep or goats dairy, or good quality meat.

Synopsis

The gut brain link is a real thing through the vagus nerve

Your gut is known as your second brain

Your gut has a large effect on your mood, energy and mental health

Taking certain foods out and adding certain foods in to your diet will go a long way to helping gut health

You are only as healthy as the foods you are able to digest and absorb

Take a good quality probiotic

Improve gut health - stay hydrated, sleep deeply, manage stress, eat slowly, eat cleaner foods

Add more fibre to your diet - i.e. berries, vegetable, seeds, nuts & oats

Supplement with a good probiotic and digestive enzyme and 3000-4000 IU of Vitamin D3 per day

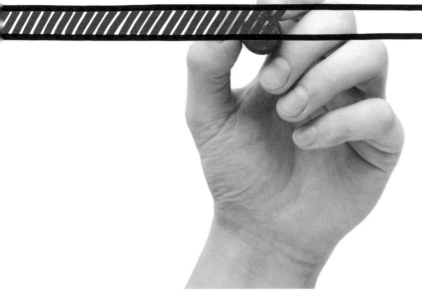

PURPOSE LOADiNG...

Fulfilling Activities, Toxicity, Habits & Closing Open Loops

How can I be more Fulfilled?

Fulfilment is something I think people often get confused with. The confusion comes with worrying about having rather than doing and just being.

When you fall into the trap of thinking you'll be happy and fulfilled when you have something or reach a certain point (weight loss?) is a fruitless path to wanting more and more. Your life certainly doesn't suddenly become more complete because you own the house or the car or reach a weight on a scales. You will soon recalibrate and want the next big thing or the next loss. Instead, why not make the weight loss happen as part of your lifestyle and include your fulfilling activities in your life to make it a low friction, long term process. Enjoy the journey not the finite destination that will not be the great thing you have cracked it up to be anyway.

Rather than rely on "things" (material goods) to be happy and fulfilled, doing things that fulfil you is a great way to start.

How do I find my fulfilling activities?

A simple exercise to figure out 21 of your fulfilling activities is this. When you talk about fulfilling activities, I don't want them to be lazy things that you haven't put any thought into. I mean things that warm you up and give you a little flutter when you think about doing it. It could be as simple as making your partner a cup of tea, to volunteering at the local soup kitchen, to a family holiday.

Write down 3 of your fulfilling activities every day for 7 days. Now these can be 5 minute activities or 2 week long activities. Don't put restrictions on them. They can be things you can incorporate into your daily, weekly, monthly or yearly life. The point is, coming away from this exercise armed with 21 things that fulfil you.

Now, let's incorporate these into your weekly schedule like you would any other appointment.

Habits

Habits are automated from behaviours we've learned from experience that have been repeated so many times it's become autonomous or automatic. Your brain learns how to respond to new situations through trial and error.

It's important to incorporate small changes you don't notice so that they go under the radar of the ego. If you make a big deal of the new habit, your ego (who hates change, remember?) will sabotage your efforts and shut it down.

You spend far more time relying on habits when stressed, tired or anxious (makes us unable to make decisions). Your brain goes into autopilot and relies on habits or behaviours we don't have to think about.

How neuro pathways work -

If you neglect a behaviour = that neuro pathway or behaviour will shrink over time
If you focus your intention and attention on a behaviour it will grow over time

Consistently doing it is the key.

New decisions are harder than old habits - pre frontal cortex gets tired, fatigue sets in, old habits kick in
The process in which habits work is like this
There's a cue i.e. walking into dark room
There's craving a change of state - Response = flicking light switch
A satisfying outcome or reward - mild comfort being able to see, light coming on

Here is another couple of examples.

> Every day
> Cue - WAKING up
> Changing state - Make coffee
> Reward - feeling alert

Exercise

> Leave running gear out the night before where you can see
> them the next morning
> Cue - Wake up - See running gear
> Reward - Feeling great afterwards

How to build Habits?

Habits are basically sub conscious behaviours we carry out as part of our day, that have deep neuro pathways that your brain uses as easy choices that expend little energy with minimal effort. You see, the brain loves low energy decision making processes. You spend roughly 45% of your time in a habitual state.

If your brain has a choice of a habit or a new behaviour, it'll choose the former every time because it's the easier of the two to carry out (remember minimal effort).

To build new habits, it's important to minimise friction between you and the new habits, and increase the friction between you and the old habits. For example, finding out the fitness class times, booking in, leaving your training clothes out for the morning so you are ready to go with less excuses available not to go.

It is also crucial that you make the cue obvious i.e. set Intentions - Class time - When - Where - What days - Book in - Attend class - Repeat

We want to increase the friction between us and our old habits. For example, this could mean getting rid of the wine in fridge on weekdays so you have to go out to get it, or hiding the remote control so you watch less TV.

The more we do it, the more natural and habitual it becomes.

So try some of these pretty interesting exercises to implement or to create the desired outcomes

1) New habit/habit stacking

So the brain releases Dopamine when doing things we enjoy right? But studies have shown that the anticipation we get from thinking about these things we enjoy give us a similar Dopamine hit. So the thought process is to try stacking a habit you like, on top of something you don't like or the new habit. If you are motivated by the reward of the thing you enjoy, this will make them more attractive which will help you stick to them. Promise yourself a reward (not food) that you will do after something you don't enjoy as much.

2) Habit of two's

When building habits, we can make them into a big deal, building them into something that becomes scary and like a massive mountain to climb. Instead, try making it a small task that you will think is doable, so you are more likely to carry it out on a more regular basis. This way, you are tricking your brain into doing an easy task that takes minimal effort, rather than talking yourself out of a big new task or habit.

So try the new habit two minute rule

Read two pages of a new book to read more

Go for a two minute run

Play the piano for two minutes

Prep a quick healthy meal

Now the reality is, you will probably spend more time doing the said new habit or activity as once you get started you will do more, but the fact is, it's the getting started that is the issue. This way we take out the friction and just do it.

We also get the satisfaction of achieving our goal of the two pages or the two minutes (we can all do two pages or two minutes right?), but you also feel amazing if you do more than what you said you would.

Building a nice positive, feel good factor around the new habit that is building momentum.

Sound good? Excellent, let's go!

3) Instant gratification

Swap the feel good factor of a takeaway with a tangible satisfaction through spending the takeaway money on something that will give you the Dopamine hit in a different way. The anticipation of a nice holiday in the sun.

So, try this. Every time you avoid takeaway or bad habit open an account and a vault on Revolut and put the exact money you would have spent on a takeaway into a holiday vault. This satisfaction will give you an immediate gratification to keep you on track and replace your takeaway craving.

How toxicity is harming me?

Your body has a threshold of toxins that it can deal with day to day. Your liver and kidneys are there to clean out and filter toxins.

Although they do a great job, if you keep putting toxins into your body at a rate that is higher than what your body can cope, your body can become toxic and with toxicity comes an opening for disease and illness to creep in as your immune system will become weak from the constant fight.

It is important to try and reduce these toxins that you are exposed to.

In this chapter we are going to go through some of the main toxins and the form they take that will resonate in your everyday life. Your liver and kidneys can tolerate a certain amount of toxins, but when you are consuming multiple times a day in different forms, that's when you should take a look at reducing some of your exposures.

Toxic forms

Food

Probably at the top of the scale of importance when it comes to reducing toxicity. We eat quite a lot each day when we add it up. Keeping foods as close to their natural state as possible is very important. Avoid the highly processed foods that have had their molecular structure changed at high heat, or additives and preservatives added that we are simply not built to consume. When you hear the word organic you might think that this is a fancy word that justifies adding euros onto anything you buy by the retail industry. But it's important we try and buy organic where possible as at least you know it's been grown naturally and responsibly and fed the right foods or not been exposed to pesticides and insecticides.

Drinks

Filtered water is for mugs, nope. I have a multiple osmotic

filter system in my kitchen so my family and I can drink clean, nonchemically treated water. I have done detailed studies on the contamination we have in our water, it's extremely common to have fluoride as a given, as well as Lead and E.coli in our tap water (amongst tonnes of other nasties).

Air fresheners/bleaches/scented cleaners

Inhaling artificially scented chemicals all day every day. No thanks. Try some essential oils like lemon and tea tree oil for an air freshener in a diffuser. This can also be used to replace household cleaning products by just adding vinegar into your spray bottle or steam cleaner. Voilà, no nasties.

People

You might not have thought of this one, but people can be toxic too. They can cause toxic stress or can be general energy suckers. This can be caused by continuous emotional abuse or accumulated burdens. Surround yourself with energy givers, mood lifters and people you aspire to be like.

Cosmetics

So many things fall into this category, including make-up, deodorant, moisturiser, sun cream, toothpaste. When you check the ingredients of these, I bet you don't recognise more than one of the ingredients. Some good replacements for toothpaste, hair gel and moisturiser can be coconut oil. When it comes to makeup, deodorant, shower gel or sun cream, try and do some research on what could be a better organic brand version.

Open loops

What is an open loop?

An Open Loop is anything pulling at your attention that doesn't belong where it is, the way it is. They can be commitments made to yourself or to another person that haven't yet been fulfilled. They can be in business as well as personal life, not necessarily tasks but any situation that is left unresolved. They can be those jobs that you've been putting off that you must do but you really can't be bothered or don't want to.

They're hanging out in limbo in your brain, they drain your mental energy without you really noticing i.e. subconsciously. Think of it like having loads of apps running in the background on your phone that use the battery without you always being aware they are open and doing so.

The main reason we find them stressful is that they are unfinished. As humans, we like to complete things, to dot the i's and cross the t's, tick the box etc. This is known as the Zeigarnik effect and it states that our minds have a natural tendency to focus on incomplete tasks. If many obligations are left unresolved in your mind, they will keep battling for your attention throughout the day and even until you go to sleep.

Having all these open loops can lead to feeling overwhelmed, which leads to stress, which means you can't concentrate on the task at hand due to knowing there are others out there.

Open loops sap mental energy (which is finite). This mental energy could be used for more important loops.

The constant pressure from open loops limits your ability to recharge when you are not at work, leaving less mental energy in the tank when you get into work mode or want to do some deep work. The loops keep building up. More to-do list tasks equals more to-do list stress.

Relationships

Which ones are life giving?

Which ones are life sucking?

It might be time to have the conversation with the life suckers to create distance. It will free up so much mental energy, or establish boundaries here too. You are not necessarily saying no to them, more like yes to you. You should never continuously leave a persona company feeling negative, drained or inadequate.

Money

Where is it going each month?

Delete monthly direct debits you are not using, check is there a better mortgage rate if you switch, can you consolidate a loan, reduce a TV or broadband bill that you've been meaning to do for months. These are draining energy and would be considered an open loop.

Home environment

What needs to be done that you've been putting off?

Room or space to de-clutter, clean, blitz, attic clear out, do up the garden?

Shelf needs fixing, freezer drawer needs replacing, these are all sapping energy subconsciously.

Free up space by booking in a time and getting it done or hire someone to do it.

Work tasks

Prioritise your 'To Do' list

Delete tasks that are no longer relevant.

Delegate jobs that are not in your remit or would be better suited to others.

Automate tasks that can be automated, there is software for EVERYTHING now that will do that annoying, time consuming.

Promises

Promised to meet an old friend, or to do them a favour? But haven't got around to it, it is draining energy. Pick up the phone and do it, you won't regret it.

Synopsis

Write down 3 fulfilling activities (all kinds/durations) every day for 7 days straight to get your 21 fulfilling

Put them in your diary each day/week/month/year

Practice to make habits stick - reduce friction of habits you want and increase friction on habits you don't

Use the new habit of 2's rule

Stack a habit you love on top of a habit you don't

Neglect old patterns of behaviour and focus on new ones you want

Reduce toxic load to perform at an optimal level

Close open loops to reduce energy loss. Split them into 4 categories - Relationships, Money, Work, Home Environment, Promises

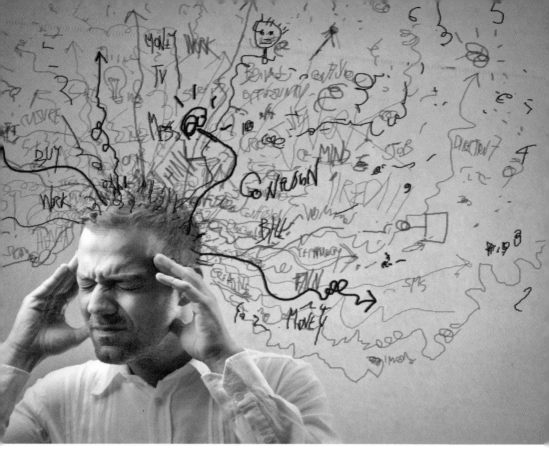

Stress

Today our lifestyle is fuelled by stress. We are running from one place to the next, eat fast food, don't value sleep and forget to breathe. We are more stressed now than ever before. In the short term stress can lead to weight gain, anxiety and sleep deprivation. In the long term, it can lead to heart attack, stroke and autoimmune diseases.

Small doses of stress can in fact be beneficial when it comes to deadlines, keeping us on our toes with things that need full attention and finding solutions in chaotic situations.

We are never going to completely alleviate stress, so importantly, we need to use tools to overcome it when we need to, and learn the difference between chronic and acute stress.

What is stress?

Our body responds to stressful situations by activation the nervous system and a cascade of hormones that help you in any given situation. I'm sure you've heard of the stories of super human strength efforts when a parent has to help their child in a life or death situation.

These specific hormones are designed to increase heart rate, metabolism and blood pressure to inhibit physical changes to help you react quickly to handle the pressure in certain stressful situations. This is known as the stress response. It is our bodies fight or flight reaction to keep us safe and alive (remember our brains main objective?). Everybody responds to events that provoke stress differently. What stresses you out, may not stress me out.

Many things may cause people to become over-stressed, including:-

- Job
- Money
- Unrealistic goals
- Over worked
- Lack of sleep
- Unhealthy relationships
- Poor communication
- Exams

- Presentations
- Public speaking

There is a difference between acute stress and chronic stress. In simple terms, acute stress is a short term stress like an exam or fight or flight situation. Chronic stress is a job, problem or relationship that causes stress every day on an ongoing basis.

The impact stress can have on you.

Stress can affect how you feel emotionally, mentally and physically. Stress can also affect how you behave.

You may feel emotionally overwhelmed, irritable and wound up. You can also feel anxious or fearful and lacking in self-esteem.

You may have difficulty concentrating and in making decisions. You may also experience racing thoughts and constant worrying.

Stress can affect you physically. You might have headaches and experience dizziness. Although you may feel tired all the time, you could have problems sleeping. Some people eat too much or too little when they are under stress. A common symptom of stress is having muscle tension or pain.

When you are experiencing stress you may find yourself drinking or smoking more than you usually do. You might snap at people for very little reason or no reason at all. Stress can make you avoid things or people you are having problems with.

What harm is stress doing?

While some of the symptoms of acute stress are fine as they are serving a purpose i.e. increase heart rate, increased blood pressure, a shot of adrenaline etc to help you deal with a physical situation, long term effects of these are not healthy and have been proven to shorten your life span through risk of heart attack and stroke to mention just a few.

How does stress make me store Fat?

Your major stress hormone Cortisol increases fat storage and blood sugars in the blood stream. This, in the short term, isn't a bad thing as your body is essentially preparing you for the fight or flight scenario. But imagine this as a chronic state for your body to be in. Increased cortisol levels in your blood promote fat storage, slowing down fat loss. It has been known to promote and accumulate fat storage around your waist. Cortisol also reduces the functions that would be deemed non-essential or detrimental in a flight or fight scenario. Even in these examples, you can see how it is important to reduce stress where possible.

How do I identify it?

Most people have experienced stress in some form, whether it be acute or chronic. Identifying what causes you stress is the first step in understanding how to cope or even better, avoid it in the future. Does stress descend on you when you meet your boss? When you think about money? When a certain time of year rolls around? Can you outsource a job you hate, address a situation you are putting on the long finger, get help from a professional to sort out a problem you can't deal with on your own? Some of these ideas can be helpful. You might be surprised at how sorting out these open loops can help save you a lot of wasted mental energy and reduce your stress.

How do I reduce it?

Managing external pressures so stressful situations don't happen to you as much. Control what you can control and don't worry about the rest.

Developing your emotional resilience so you're better at coping with tough situations when they do happen and don't feel quite so stressed.

The Complete Morning Rituals™

Changing the way you wake up in the morning has the potential to set you up for the day ahead, and to be able to help you deal with your days' stressors in a far more controlled and grounded manner. Instead of checking your phone first thing and being accessible, try the three techniques below that will keep you more grounded, more relaxed and emotionally stable before you let the days' stresses set in.

Breath work - Changing your state through oxygenating your brain and grounding yourself first thing in the morning is one of the most effective ways of making you less stressed and effected by what life is likely to throw at you throughout the day. Simply spend 10 Minutes breathing through your nose. Close your mouth and breath through your tummy, relax your chest.

How to - Breath in through the nose, out through the nose for 3-5 seconds each. Just count and breath.

Move - Change your physiology through movement, it doesn't have to be anything big, just walk, some squats, plank, some press ups to get the blood moving, the endorphins rushing around your body and the feel good factor into your morning.

How to - Move your body. Try this - 10 Jumping Jacks - 10 Press ups - 10 Squats - 10 Second Plank x 2 Sets

Journal - Change your mood from anxious or stressed to grateful. It's not possible to feel both. Simply write down the 3-5 things you are grateful for in your life. Kids, family, work, relationships, health, a roof over your head etc. Your brain cannot be both stressed/anxious and grateful at the same time. You'd prefer to be grateful, right?

How to - Write down 3-5 things you are grateful for every morning and/or evening.

Synopsis

Acute stress is ok, chronic is not

Acute stress can be very beneficial in terms of helping you in stressful situations

Stress can cause your body to store fat around the stomach area

Identifying what stresses you out is crucial before trying to alleviate it

Stress increase risks of stroke, heart and reduced life span

Reduce stress through breathing, journaling, exercising

Supplement with Vit c (3-5grams per day) to reduce stress

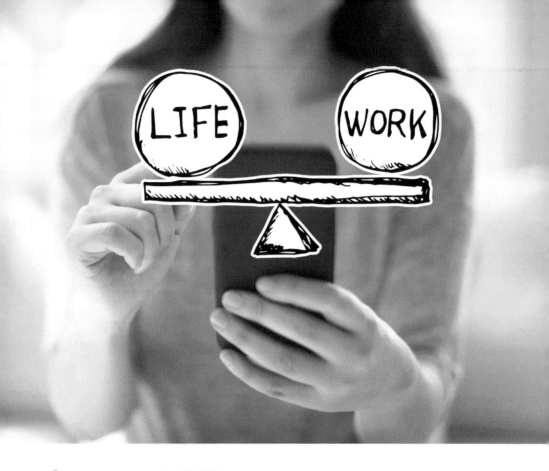

Life Work Balance
Why should I have a better balance?

The majority of people I come in contact with are stressed, are anxious, are worried and feel like they need to do better and to be better, but are going about it the wrong way. Working harder and for longer is not the way to progress in life, in my opinion.

Having less time with your family, more time in front of a screen, or more time sitting are all unnatural things that we were not built to do.

Having a more balanced approach to your life can be easier than you think, but only by flipping your priorities on their head. For example, what do you value more, yourself, your work, your family or your self-development? For the most part you are going to say your family, but do they come first in reality or do you sacrifice quality time because you think it will benefit them long term. Maybe...but I know for one thing, that spending quality time with them now will certainly benefit them and you RIGHT NOW.

The thought process of planning for the future is important. Working your fingers to the bone now for the future and putting all your eggs in that basket is a flawed plan. You need to learn to have the balance that will create a more enjoyable journey because you never know what will happen in the future. Plan for the future but enjoy the now. That is what we are going to help you work out now in this chapter.

Who Is the most important person in your life?

Why do you put yourself bottom of the pile? Last to look after yourself, last to put time and investment into yourself? The famous Tony Robbins saying, on an aircraft, be the first to put the oxygen mask on yourself so you can then help others, as you are the most important person in your life and you should put yourself first to help others. It's not selfish, it's selfless, as no one else will probably notice that you have put yourself first, and if they aren't happy with that, maybe they don't have your best interests at heart.

Imagine right now sitting reading this, how much your life would be enhanced if you put yourself first for once and invested in yourself in terms of getting healthier, happier, more relaxed, more content and self-confident.

Who will it benefit?

When you think about it, who will actually benefit from you putting yourself first and becoming a happier healthier person? Who do you come in contact with on a regular basis? More than likely they will.

They will notice you being happier and healthier, anyone who cares about you will be delighted as they will want to see you happy right?

Who would benefit from you being more productive, having bucket loads of energy, a more positive outlook on life, more confidence, more mental clarity, focus and drive?

By adding a better balance to your life, it will lead to you being a better brother, sister, husband, wife, son, daughter, cousin, grandparent, grandchild (you get the picture). You are literally going to be a rebooted, upgraded version of yourself, that will enhance every aspect of your life.

How can I balance my life & work better?

You can balance by having a formula that will break up your days and weeks into a framework that will help you give time to each part of your life that will help.

But first we need to figure out what it is you value and what your values are.

Ok let's dive in.

Write down the 4 things in order of priority that you value in your life

_____

_____

_____

_____

Write down the 4 values you aspire to live by

_____

_____

_____

_____

You need to bear in mind when you talk about your lifestyle balance, what you have written down in terms of your values and their alignment with what you actually value.

The Complete Balance Formula™

Now we are going to split the main aspects of your life into 4 quadrants.

Work - How can we enhance your work performance and reduce your work load through Deleting/Prioritising/Delegating/Automating your workload?

Family - How can we spend more QUALITY time with family/friends/kids/spouse etc each week? Put it in the diary like you would any other appointment.

Health - How can we prioritise this part of our life, because if we don't have this, we have nothing. Put it in the diary like you would any other appointment.

Self-development - What haven't we done that we've been meaning to? maybe do a course, listen to more podcasts, read more books, learn an instrument or language or just breath work and daily cold water therapy. Put it in the diary like you would any other appointment.

By writing down your values and then putting a structure to it, you should now be able to plan your week a little better with more balance and acknowledgement of what is actually important to you in your life.

I see so many people living a miserable life in the hope that it will magically be amazing once they can afford to retire when they are 65. You more than likely aren't going to be able to physically do what you can now when you are 65 years old, so why wait to enjoy your life? Plan for the future (think outside the box) but enjoy the now and spend money on things you enjoy, that enhance and give you the best chance to prolong your life in the best way possible.

Synopsis

Prioritise "YOU" as number one for a more balanced life

It will benefit those close to you more than you realise

Write down 4 things that you value in your life

Write down 4 values you like to live by

Split your life into 4 parts - Health/Family/Work/Self Development and make time for each

Work on each part and book them into your diary like any other appointment

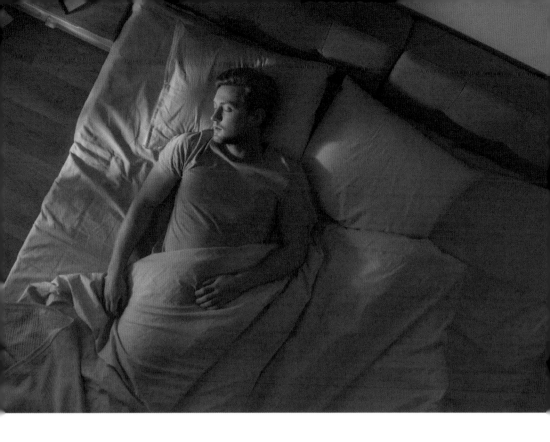

Sleep
How important is sleep?

Sleep, is without doubt, the most under-valued piece of the health and wellness jigsaw. It is for the most part viewed as an after-thought. The reality is, if you get your sleep right, most of the other parts of your life will slip into place far more easily.

Some fascinating sleep insights:-

- 1 in 3 people don't get enough sleep

- Sleep is the number one foundation of which
  holistic health sits

- Shorter your Sleep = Shorter Your Life

- Average sleep time for the world's population is 6 hours and
  30 minutes (Recommended 7-9 hours)

"If you are deprived of sleep (5-6 hours per night), you can consume,
on average an extra 200-300 calories per day. Leptin decreases, your
satiety hormone (telling you, you are full) & ghrelin hormone
increases (telling you, you are hungry)"

Professor Matthew Walker

Why we sleep?

Sleep is a naturally recurring state of mind and body. Without
sleep, we would simply not survive. Sleep restores the nervous,
skeletal, and muscular systems. It's a vital process that maintains
mood, memory, and cognitive function. It plays a large role in the
function of the Endocrine system (Produces Hormones) including
regulating hunger and satiety hormones. It also restores the
Immune system (protects against disease/heals/helps you recover
from illness).

One night with lack of sleep can make us as insulin resistant as a
type 2 diabetic

What are the stages of sleep?

Light sleep - The stage in between full consciousness & deep
sleep. This is approximately 50% of your night's sleep.

Deep sleep - This is the restorative sleep stage (first half of night's sleep). It is approximately 25% of your night's sleep. It tends to decline with age. Most of your growth hormone is produced at this stage (recovery, muscle building etc.)

Dream sleep (REM) - This is the stage when brain activity is similar to when awake. This equates to approximately 25% of your night's sleep. You get into Dream sleep stage 4-5 times per night. It helps to regulate body temperature and is most likely when you experience dreams. It is also when your body recovers emotionally..

94% of couples who sleep in contact are happier in their relationship.

How to get better sleep?

- No Caffeine After 1pm. It stays in your system for 6-7 hours and can be like supping an espresso before bed when you have a coffee after lunch.

- Alcohol inhibits the emotional part of your brains recovery. If you are drinking multiple times a week, your ability to recover fully on an emotional level is compromised.

- No Phones/Computer (blue Light) two hours before bed. The light stimulates the hormone melatonin that tells your brain to be awake as it sees light and assumes it's day time.

- Magnesium therapy (Hot Bath/Tablets/Spray). This helps your muscles unwind, recover and relax.

- Essential oils on your pillow. Lavender can help you unwind and relax into a deeper sleep.

- Brain Dump in your Journal/Share Wins/Gratitude/Breath

Work. When you are struggling to unwind and your brain is active, simple exercises such as journaling, or brain dumping can help offload what's on your mind down onto paper. You can include what is on your mind, what you have to do the next day, what your wins are for the day, what you are grateful for.

- Workout/Exercise (Not Too Late). Helping expend excess energy is a very effective way of improving sleep. Releasing endorphins as we have discussed in previous chapters, has massive benefits from clearing your head and tiring you out to helping you sleep better.

- Sleep in a dark room/comfortable bed. This might sound simple, but is your room dark? Have you invested in a comfortable bed? Remember you spend most of your time in your shoes or in your bed, invest in both.

Surgeons awake for more than 24 hours take 14% longer to carry out tasks & make 20% more mistakes

What's my ideal sleep routine?

Aim to get up at the same time every day. Try not to vary this even at the weekend. It's easy to fall into the trap of having a lie in. Pair this with later bed times, it can cause social jet lag. This just means your body clock is adjusting to a different routine at the weekend, than on weekdays. You feel tired because you are having to readjust to a different routine, causing tiredness, irritability and experiencing the Monday Blues.

You shouldn't be getting afternoon slumps. The food you are eating daily can massively contribute to this. If you have addressed the diet part, then sleep is most likely the issue.

So we've established getting out of bed at the same time each day is important. Now try and get to bed 15 mins earlier each night until you don't get an afternoon slump.

Very simply repeat this until you feel energised through-out the day.

Sex drive is determined by sleep depth and quality. For every extra hour, 14% Increase of likely hood of increased libido

Synopsis

Aim to sleep for 7-9 hours

Aim for quality as much as quantity

Watch your holistic health skyrocket if you work on both

It will be far easier to exercise and eat more healthily if you have enough sleep

Your hormones will be more balanced

Stay healthier and recover quicker

Ultimately live longer

Use Zinc (10-14mg)/Magnesium (320mg- 420mg) before bed

Use a few drops of pure lavender essential oil on your pillow

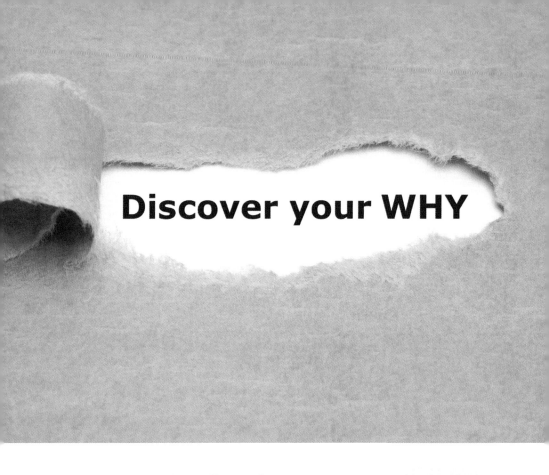

Your Why - Motivations

Before you start the journey to change, understanding what your main purpose, or reason to change is crucial to the level of success you will achieve. You can set all the goals you like but until you understand why you are really doing something, on the deepest level, you can easily drift and be like a GPS navigation system with no end destination.

What do you really want?

So what is it you want to happen as an end result when embarking on your new journey?

_____

_____

_____

Get specific, I don't mean the generic "I want to tone up, lose weight" blah blah. I mean what is it you really want on a deeper level?

What it actually is you want to achieve i.e. I would like to drop 3 clothes sizes, 30lbs of body fat, fit into that dress/shirt that's been sitting in my wardrobe comfortably in the next 6 months.

Why do you really want it?

Finding that "WHY" on the deepest level you can find, will help you when times are tough and you need to find motivation from within. So what's the reason why?

- To be more attractive or reconnect with your partner?
- To fall in love with what you see in the mirror again?
- Be confident and proud walking down the beach in your swim suit?
- Get your mojo back when naked again?
- To be there for you kids and show them the way forward because it's your duty?

1 _____

2 _____

3 _____

4 _____

Motivations

Struggling with motivation is a tough one. It's one of the most common struggles when it comes to being consistent. Working on the basis of my four pillars of motivation will help you massively overcome this.

Whatever it may be, think about it and take the time to write it down. As Tony Robbins says; "If you do that, It becomes real and it is far more likely to happen."

Here is a pretty cool way of working your "Why's" out, by figuring out what your motivating factors are.

The four pillars of motivation are:

Internal motivation

What's in it for me?

_____

External motivation

Who will benefit around me from me being happier and healthier?

Security motivation

What would I possibly lose if I don't do something ASAP?

_____

Opportunity motivation

What opportunities will present themselves if I get to my target weight/more energy/inches loss/more confident self etc?

_____

When do you want It by?

Putting an end date on things will make it something to strive for. A good way of working out a time frame for what you want to achieve (like I did for this book) is to reverse engineer it. So, how much can you commit to making progress on your journey each day, each week, each month? Work out what's realistically doable (Ask a professional if you don't know). Then work backwards from your end-goal. Put it in the diary and tell people so you are accountable. Or be accountable to a coach who can get you there quicker.

_____

What do you need to do to get it?

What is it you need to do in terms of actionable behaviours and habits each day that are going to get you closer in small steps each day. Workout, Drink more water?

_____

Who do you need to be to get it?

At the moment, you are reading this because you would like to change something in your life for the better. Who you are and how you behave will need to be different for you to make the required changes. We all know what doing the same thing over and over again and expecting different results means.

Identifying the roadblocks that are stopping you in your head is the best place to start.

Why have you not been able to achieve these changes in the past?

How do we remove the blockages?

What behaviours have you identified that need to change to reach the goals you set earlier? Sleep better, make better food choices? Find something you enjoy doing or join a community that exercise - this will help your consistency!

What are your desired outcomes

Putting all of this together can be tough, but a simple process will help you in terms of clarity and focus. So let's go.

So let's get clear, what do you want to happen in the next

- 12 Months?
- 6 months?
- 3 months?

So you might be wondering why I've put the time frames back to front. Well I find reverse engineering things will help with the step by step process.

What do you want to achieve as your long term goal, let's say in 12 months?

Action Step 1: _____

Action Step 2: _____

Action Step 3: _____

What do you want to achieve as your medium term goal, let's say 6 months?

Action Step 1: _____

Action Step 2: _____

Action Step 3: _____

What do you want to achieve as your short term goal, let's say 3 months?

Action Step 1: _____

Action Step 2: _____

Action Step 3: _____

The point is, building behaviours and habits that will serve you better is key to achieving long term and sustainable results.

Building habits

Step 1) Apply the rule of twos' to your new desired habits. Make it small and easy to achieve initially.

- Read two pages of a self-help book

- Run for 2 mins
- Workout for 2 mins

Step 2) Habit stacking

Stack a habit or activity you love doing, on top of a habit you are trying to introduce. The anticipation and dopamine hit of looking forward to the habit you love will help you do the habit before it. Do the new habit and then reward yourself with the habit you love.

Are your habits and outcomes aligned?

It's all well and good setting your ideal outcomes but without looking into your current habits and making sure they are aligned, things will fail, and fast.

Wanting to lose 2 stones in 6 months without changing your dietary habits isn't going to happen. What has got you to this place in your life has been because of the choices, actions and habits you have consistently carried out on a daily basis.

I use weight loss as an example, as that is most likely one of the key components of you wanting to choose healthier habits and lifestyle.

So if your goal is to achieve a two stone weight loss in 6 months, learning what calories you need to be consuming to be in a calorie deficit, figuring out what foods are going to nourish you and what format you are going to consume those calories in, is vital for your success. PREP IS KEY. Knowing what you are going to eat and when is so important for you to consistently get results. Letting yourself get hungry with no healthy options to eat is a fast track road to failure. Plan your meals ahead methodically and precisely and this will be a smooth and easy process.

Synopsis

Work out what you want

Work out who you need to become to get it

Work out what you need to do to get it

When you want it by

Figure out your 4 pillars of motivation

What is the big outcome?

What small habits do you want to build daily to change?

These habits and outcomes need to be aligned

Conclusion

Having consumed the content of the book, I hope you found it interesting, insightful and implementable. I have tried to put it in as simple terms as possible, exactly like I like to learn. If you implement this information, it will change your life for the better. But the problem is rarely information, it's the implementation of the information.

What will hold you back from putting this all together is most likely one or two of the following:-

1) Overwhelm - This can be extremely debilitating. When you take on too much information without the structure to put it together.

2) You tell yourself the same old story that you can't do it. Change the story you tell yourself.

3) You have no one to help support you and keep you accountable to implement.

Which one sounds like it may impact you?

Our Complete 90 Day Body & Mindset program will give you a step by step process of how to put this together over the next 90 days and beyond. Weekly tasks, weekly calls, daily workouts and nutrition plans and seminars to help you implement and lose up to 2 stone and drop two clothes sizes in just 90 days. This can be done remotely, in private one to one or in a small group format setting.

At your fingertips, you have some seriously powerful information. It would be a terrible waste just to sit on it and keep struggling on your health and fitness journey.

Please go to **www.completepersonaltraining.ie** and apply for a complimentary consultation, where we will work out where you are now on your health and fitness journey, where you would like to get to and build a plan for you to do so in the most sustainable and direct route possible.

Let's make this time different from anything you've tried in the past. You know now, through reading this book, why you have not been successful and yo-yo'd with your weight in the past. Now, let me help you implement a proven process so you never have to struggle with diets again.

"Master your mindset and never diet again"

Our immersive luxury retreats offer you 7 nights of luxury in our mega villa in Lanzarote. We whisk you away to the sun drenched island to immerse yourself in a constant state of growth, learning and fun. Our Complete Mind & Body Retreat to Lanzarote will teach you how to cook and eat healthily, we have daily workouts, morning yoga and afternoon massages to treat every aspect of your health and wellness. In the mornings we have fascinating, inclusive and enjoyable excursions including luxury boat charters, kayaking, stand up paddleboarding, volcano treks, market visits, scuba diving and much more. Our evening life coaching modules will open your eyes to a new way of thinking and living.

You will return home having built a clear plan of action and full set of goals to achieve on returning home.

You will return home having built a clear plan of action and full set of goals to achieve on returning home.

You will have new direction, a new lust for life and it is just the reset and kickstart you may need to get you going on your health and fitness journey.

Please go to **www.competetransformationretreats.ie** for more information on our upcoming retreats.

"Never worry about being unmotivated again"

What we do

Complete Personal Training & Complete Transformation Retreats are primarily a semi-private or private personal training, results driven business focusing on mindset, fitness, nutrition and luxury foreign retreats abroad.

We motivate people just like you, who may be stuck in a rut, or have lost motivation through neuroscience, education and support to make sure you get guaranteed results fast.

"My experience diving deep into personality types and your likely trajectory is crucial in helping communicate successfully with my clients on the deepest level."

As your holistic health is our priority, we give you clear direction and we support you through the process, wrapping our team around you and holding your hand through the tough times.

"Being able to deliver information in certain ways to each individual personality type helps me reach them in the most powerful way possible to successfully effect change"

The programs we offer provide accountability and support with a close-knit fitness family environment to help you get started, whatever your fitness level, without the intimidation of a standard gym.

The three main aspects we focus on in our Complete 90 Day Body & Mindset Matrix™ program include -

Our Complete Nutrition System™ helps reduce inflammation, bloating and water retention, while tightening loose skin and sky-rocketing your fat loss results.

The Complete Afterburn Workouts™ will building lean athletic muscle and torch body fat, while cranking up your metabolism like a fat burning furnace for up to 36 hours after your workout.

The Complete Mindset Matrix™ will help build lean athletic muscle and torch body fat, while cranking up your metabolism like a fat burning furnace for up to 36 hours after your workout.

Complete Sleep Formula Seminar™ Sleep underpins every part of your health and is vastly underestimated when it comes to mastering your overall health.

We train everyone, from busy professionals, celebrities and burnt-out parents, to athletes and the younger generation who need guidance and coping mechanisms as they may have lost their way. The Complete System really will change your life.

What are some of our life coaching modules we run on retreat?

The Complete Nutrition System™

Learn our unique anti-inflammatory eating plan that aims for long term optimal health and nourishes your body to perform as the best version of you.

The Complete Morning Rituals™

Start the day free of stress and anxiety and be fully bulletproof.

The Complete Goal Focus™

Add complete direction to your life with a different spin.

The Complete Stress Solution™

Identify and deal with stress the right way.

The Complete Life Work Balance™

How to live a more fulfilled and balanced life.

The Complete Mindset Matrix™

Learn how the mind works and how our 4 pillars can help transform your mindset, from bogged down and frustrated, to free and happy.

The Complete Sleep Formula™

Sleep underpins how you perform during the day. Learn how to sleep more deeply to super charge your energy levels.

A special thank you to:-

Ian Johnston for book design, guidance, formatting and help self-publishing

Eibhlin Johnston for proof reading and advice

James O'Reilly for cover photos

Barry Sheehan for cover design

Paul Hatton for proof reading

Printed in Great Britain
by Amazon

20601519R00054